The Problem with Paleo

Taking a Deeper Look at the Popular Myths and Fallacies of Eating Like a Caveman

By: Joey Lott

www.joeylotthealth.com

2

Publishing services provided by 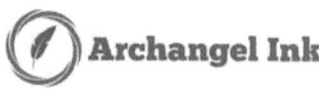 Archangel Ink

ISBN: 1517511682
ISBN-13: 978-1517511685

Table of Contents

4

I Got Paleoed

This is a book that intends to refute the paleo diet fallacy. My hope is not to convert you to my way of seeing things or to join my diet cult. I have no such cult. I don't care how you eat or what you believe. That is your business. However, if you feel trapped or unwell in your dietary dogma, my intention with this book is to offer you a way out of that trap—a way to begin to trust in the innate intelligence of your body and to begin to treat your body with kindness and humility rather than being the dietary dictator that paleo (and other restrictive dietary ideologies) tends to turn us into in some form or another.

This book isn't really about me or my story as much as it is an invitation to explore and question the commonly held truths of paleo dieters. However, I chose to write this book because I have personal experience with the dangers and pitfalls of paleo rigidity and the pursuit of dietary (and health) perfection. So to begin with, I'd like to share with you my own introduction to paleo as well as some of the hijinks that ensued so that, perhaps, you can see some of your own story in mine.

The paleo diet is reportedly the fastest growing trend today. And if popular Google searches or threads on marksdailyapple.com are any indication, some of the most common reasons people are interested in the paleo diet involve a desire to lose weight, get "in shape," and "cure" or prevent conditions like diabetes and cardiovascular disease.

My introduction to the so-called paleo diet was different than most people because I wasn't trying to cure myself of diabetes nor was I interested in losing weight. In fact, when I first started eating according to the paleo diet principles, I was already severely underweight.

In order for you to fully appreciate my introduction to the paleo diet, I'm going to need to give you a little bit of backstory to offer some context. I had been a committed vegan for the better part of seventeen years, but I had grown disillusioned. My years as a vegan were characterized by an unhealthy obsession with food and then an increasingly unhealthy obsession with just about everything else. I had grown extremely anxious and compulsive to the point where I was unable to function very well.

In 2009, I reached a breaking point. I felt desperate for a positive change in my life, but frankly, I was willing to gamble on *any* change. I had tried many different options—changing coasts, then countries, getting married, getting divorced, psychedelics, a *very* short stint at an ashram, and more—so you'll perhaps understand that my choice, as strange as it was, came at the end of a long search for *something* to help.

In October of 2009, the lease on my apartment ran out. I decided not to renew. I took a leave of absence from my business, and I drove to northern Wisconsin to spend the winter living outside in the woods with a group from a wilderness school. It's the sort of place that appeals mostly to middle-class, white Americans and Europeans who are frustrated with the guilt and discomfort of their all-too-comfortable lives, which leave them feeling isolated from the pulse of life. So instead, they go get uncomfortable for a while.

Part of being uncomfortable, apart from sleeping outside in 30-below-zero temperatures and having no central heat, also involved giving up control over entertainment as well as *food*. We were never deprived, since the school provided ample food. However, the fare was designed to mimic the food of the native people of Wisconsin—you know, before they were cheeseheads. So we ate lots of deer, bear, beaver, raccoon, and fish from the local lakes. We also ate dried wild edibles that had been gathered by some of the residents during the green season such as nettles, wild leeks, and tamarack leaves. We also ate cultivated vegetables, predominantly cabbage.

On the one hand, after my years of veganism, eating meat and animal fat once again was deeply nourishing. However, the low-carbohydrate nature of the diet produced worsening emaciation in my case. The cold nights became something that I dreaded; despite the fact that my sleeping bags were rated to 60 below and I had ample padding beneath me, I was so cold at night that my sleep was horrible. This despite the fact that I was eating like it was going out of style. I was gorging on fat, meat, and vegetables, and though there were no scales or nutrition labels in the woods, I estimate that I was eating 4000 calories a day *and still losing weight.*

There were many things I didn't like about my stay at the wilderness school, but there was much that I did like. It was beautiful and intimate and close in a way I had never experienced. Much of the fear I had of living without comforts fell away, and I found a new confidence that I had not known previously. So after I left, I was convinced that I wanted to continue to live in a way that supported much of the good that I experienced while there.

Among the many things that I took away from the experience was paleo. Granted, I felt terrible, weak, and anxious eating that way, but I also felt a nourishment that I hadn't felt in a long time (with veganism), and that appealed to me.

Perhaps a year afterward, I found *The Primal Blueprint* by Mark Sisson, which is, along with Chris Kresser's and Robb Wolf's books, one of the most popular books on "paleo." Sisson differentiates "primal" from "paleo" by supposedly taking a more progressive, open-minded view of health and nutrition than paleo. But ultimately, he makes a stronger case against grains, dairy, and *carbohydrates* than just about anyone else.

After reading Sisson's book, I was convinced that my health problems were due to my lack of strict adherence to a "pure" paleo (primal) diet. At the time, I was extremely fatigued to the point where I was struggling even to walk. Needless to say, lifting heavy things and sprinting like Sisson's beloved Grok supposedly would have was out of the question. But I thought that might have been due to the fact that I had slipped up by introducing dairy into my diet; at the time, I was struggling to eat enough calories, and so I was eating cottage cheese and massive amounts of cream. But after I read *The Primal Blueprint,* I decided to stop eating any dairy in hopes it would help me to feel better. Instead, I started waking up in the middle of the night with extreme nausea followed by violent diarrhea and/or vomiting. At the time, I thought maybe it was a dairy "detox," and I vowed never to eat dairy again since clearly it produced horrible toxic withdrawal reactions.

It took another year of trying to do paleo "right" before I finally gave up. In the month before giving up, I had been eating little more than eggs, gelatinous cuts of grass-fed beef and lamb, lots of bone broth and offal, and lots of non-starchy vegetables and herbs. I felt worse and worse, and so just before I quit, I made a last-ditch effort by following the so-called autoimmune paleo protocol. Once I recovered from the bout of kidney stones I experienced while involved in the autoimmune shenanigans, I asked the question, "What would Grok do?" and decided that if starving Grok had had access to potatoes, butter, sugar, maple syrup, and white rice, he would have eaten that stuff to restore his health.

Okay, I didn't *really* ask, "What would Grok do?" because frankly, that would be weird. But I did decide that's what *I* would do under those circumstances. I hadn't eaten sugar, maple syrup, or white rice in decades. In fact, I had been afraid of them. Terrified, even. And unlike other people who have reported their paleo failures due to irresistible cravings for cake, ice cream, and bread, I had no such cravings. In fact, I had no appetite. I don't particularly like sweet things nor do I particularly like bread or cake. But I felt that these foods were necessary in order to restore health to my body, so despite my fears and ideology, I started eating outside of the paleo-approved foods—not only that, but well outside of the foods that are generally accepted as healthy. And based on the research that I have done since, much of which I have written about in other books such as *Hungry*, I now know that that was the right thing to do. I had been blinded by an ideology.

Subsequently, my health improved dramatically. I still ate meat, eggs, and non-starchy vegetables, but I also started eating dairy, sugar, bread, potatoes, pasta, and lots of other stuff that is generally off limits according to paleo guidelines. I reconsidered my whole nutritional worldview and began to research these matters to see how the heck I had been so mistaken.

I know I'm not the only one. Sisson's website, marksdailyapple.com, boasts 400,000 subscribers, and combined, the most popular paleo diet books have sold millions of copies. Whether we call it paleo or primal or the caveman diet or NeanderThin or any other such nonsense, it's moved away from the fringe and toward the mainstream. And surely, for some people it works just fine. Many people are probably able to experience good health balanced with a *moderate* approach to a so-called paleo lifestyle; they follow the 80/20 rule—or maybe 70/30 or perhaps 50/50—improving their health by reducing their visits to McDonald's, increasing their intake of grass-fed meat, enjoying a greater variety of vegetables, eating sufficient carbohydrates, and moving in healthier ways (i.e., avoiding sedentarism *and* chronic cardio). However, I know I'm not the only one who took it too far and turned it into an eating disorder, doing injury to myself in my zealotry. So this book is for those of you who need a voice of reason, gentleness, sanity, and nourishment to call you back to health and balance.

In this book, I will expose the fallacy of paleo and invite you to allow balance into your life if you've taken the paleo ideology to the extreme. The key word is "balance" because I am not asking you nor inviting you to swing to another extreme and forego any benefits that may be derived from your experiments with paleo. There is good to be had from those experiments, and we'll discuss some of that as we explore together. However, the reality is that if paleo—or the version of paleo that you have tried to make work—hasn't worked for you, it may be that it just doesn't work for you. And that's okay. It doesn't mean you're a failure. Nor does it mean that you're doomed to develop diabetes, cardiovascular disease, cancer, and Alzheimer's just because you aren't living like an imaginary Grok. It turns out that paleo doesn't actually offer the insurance that advocates claim, and plenty of people are healthy even though they eat dairy and wheat and sugar. Heck, there are even healthy people who drink Coca-Cola made with high-fructose corn syrup and Twinkies made from...well, I have no idea what Twinkies are made from!

Despite the fact that consuming *lots* of sugar, white rice, and pasta turned out to be very beneficial for me in rediscovering health, I don't have a huge appetite for them in general. So while I was initially drinking milkshakes with *obscene* amounts of sugar in them, I've since toned that down quite a bit, and after an initial recovery period, I now eat a fairly "balanced" diet that includes plenty of paleo-approved foods such as eggs, gelatinous meats, herbs, sweet potatoes, beets, carrots, onions, and so forth. And, I don't tend to eat a *whole* lot of grain simply because I don't have a strong desire for it, though frankly, I do go through phases when I enjoy me some heaping bowls of rice or pasta with lots of butter and maybe some cheese.. But I *do* eat a *lot* of potatoes, cheese, butter, and milk, and I do drink quite a lot of fruit juice, and I eat sugar for therapeutic effect if and when I feel that it would be helpful. Why? Because I have found that eating what I desire or what my body feels that it needs tends to be much more healthful than eating what I *think* I should eat. Oh, and it's a heck of a lot *easier* and *more enjoyable* than being so rigid and restrictive.

The reason I mention what I eat these days isn't to suggest that it is important. Rather, I just want to make the point that in many ways, my present diet isn't terribly at odds with paleo ideals. Sure, paleo *usually* frowns upon dairy and potatoes, and grains and sugar are almost always out. But I am not coming at this discussion with a strong bias that grains are essential to health or that we *need* chocolate cake or Lifesavers or Snickers. I live fairly simply and have simple tastes. That's just my preference. I actually prefer simple tastes to complex tastes *most* of the time. For example, a hash brown made with just potato, butter, and salt is, to me, a nearly perfect food. Granted, a bit of melted cheese on top is pretty good too. I'm not precisely *anti*-paleo. I just *question* the rigidity and zeal with which it is often pursued and promoted. In fact, it often has a sort of religious tone to it, and like all religion, it is worth questioning if one feels trapped or harmed by it in any way.

Hopefully I've already made this clear, but just in case I haven't, let me state emphatically that I have no beef with anyone eating in whatever way makes them feel good. I have no new, better diet to sell you, and I don't need your support or agreement for my choices. If paleo is working for you, then that is wonderful, and more power to you. But if it isn't—and I mean if it isn't working in *any* way, including physically, emotionally, psychologically, or otherwise—then let's explore together. Maybe you'll discover that paleo isn't really the Holy Grail you'd imagined it to be and that it's okay to let go.

I am well aware that there are many variations on the paleo diet. Some are far more lenient than others while some are ultra-restrictive. And yes, I am aware that paleo isn't strictly synonymous with low carbohydrate. However, in many cases, paleo *is* ultra-restrictive in practical terms, and in many cases, it really *is* synonymous with low carbohydrate. And in any case, finally, the question becomes, "Why are we so interested in any sort of special diet at all?" Is our search for the right diet all that different than the search for the right religion in hopes that we'll discover salvation and never have to experience sickness or discomfort? Maybe, as an added bonus, we might get to look down our noses smugly at others who aren't so perfect?

In this book, we'll explore some of the claims, beliefs, and practices that are common in the "paleosphere." So yeah, some of what I'll refute in this book isn't what is advocated by *everyone* who promotes paleo. So don't get your loincloth all bunched up just because I argue the fallacies of low-carbohydrate diets while not *all* paleo diets are explicitly low carbohydrate. Enough *are* that it's important to refute. And, don't worry, there's something here for everyone. Let's dig in.

The Premise of Paleo

Whether we're talking about Cordain's paleo, Wolf's paleo, Sisson's primal, or any other variation, the essential premise remains very similar. The basic idea is that about 10,000 years ago when humans are thought to have first adopted agricultural practices on a large scale—at the advent of the Neolithic period—human health took a nosedive, and we saw the beginning of the rise of the diseases of civilization. The belief is that prior to that, our hunter-gatherer ancestors were healthy and happy in every way. Therefore, we are told that if we emulate what our Paleolithic ancestors did—and especially what they *ate*—we can escape the fate of the majority of modern humans and live happily and healthfully, remaining flexible, strong, and active until we are 100, at which point we might die peacefully in our sleep.

We're told that the *foods* of the Neolithic era are at fault for all of the health problems that are rampant today such as diabetes, cardiovascular disease, Alzheimer's, Parkinson's, and cancer. And if you feel that you are overweight, you're told that it's all those nasty Neolithic foods that are inflating your waistline. Plus, we're told that lots of other health problems are also easily pinned on those same foods—problems like insomnia, arthritis, osteoporosis, and so on.

What are the Neolithic foods that are said to be causing the problems? Well, not Neolithic foods like broccoli, apples, carrots, and almonds. Rather, it's a specific subset of Neolithic foods that are said to be at fault—namely dairy, sugar, grains, and legumes.

That's it in a nutshell. And it's a nice story. After all, we hear about the so-called obesity epidemic and that 1 in 7 men will develop prostate cancer or that 1 in 4 deaths are caused by cardiovascular disease, and we want to find the way to protect ourselves, to stay healthy. The paleo promise tells us that our Paleolithic ancestors who never ate dairy, sugar, grain, or legumes had no such conditions or diseases. We are told that they were trim, fit, and healthy. So we are led to believe that *if only we will eat like they did*, we too will experience radiant health and vitality now and forever.

And, to be certain, for some people, it *seems* to improve health, at least for a while. Many people report experiencing more energy, improved mood, and better vitality when switching to a paleo diet. But is that *because* of the paleo diet? And will a paleo diet make good on its promise as true life insurance?

The Switch

Many of the most inspiring paleo "success" stories are the ones with dramatic health improvements. Many of us have read the case studies or watched the videos in which we witness remarkable transformations; some report that they have experienced "miracle healings" as a result of transitioning to a paleo diet—though, to be perfectly frank, most of the transformations are weight loss, and while some of it appears healthy, a lot of it does not. In other words, paleo is sometimes the next phase of disordered, restrictive eating that leads to unhealthy weight loss. I have seen profiles of paleo weight loss promoted on the websites of popular paleo gurus in which the "before" photos looked healthy and the "after" photos looked skeletal. That really ought to raise some concern about the level-headedness of the paleo advocates. They aren't seeing clearly.

But the question that begs to be asked is, are these transformations due to some miracle of paleo or are they merely the result of a person's dedication to making what they perceive to be a positive change? There's a phenomenon known as the placebo effect, which means that if someone expects to experience a particular effect or benefit, then he or she may experience that effect despite the fact that the treatment is a sham. This is such a powerful phenomenon that well-designed studies have to control for it. I can't help but notice that in almost every case, these transformation stories have common characteristics. Namely, the people who are transforming have a *desire and intention* to transform. That is powerful. And not only do they have a desire and intention to transform, they also take steps *beyond a change in diet* to bring about these desired changes. In other words, some of the "miracle transformations" are from people who not only cut out sugar and grain from their diets, but also start lifting weights, giving priority to sleep, and finding healthier social outlets.

Perhaps most significant is that the transition to paleo often brings about a new and more balanced awareness of nutrition. If someone was drinking Big Gulps and snacking on Twinkies before the transition to paleo and then suddenly commits to eating meat, fruit, and vegetables instead because they perceive that it is healthier, it shouldn't be surprising to see a transformation. But then again, similar transformations are seen when people transition to a whole food vegan diet from, say, a regular diet of McDonald's. Does that mean that veganism is healthy in the long term? Not necessarily. Does that mean that veganism is the ultimate diet? Nope. It just means that it was a relative improvement. Interestingly, those who switch to a paleo diet from a long-term vegan diet may experience benefits, but does that mean that paleo is the ultimate diet? No, it does not. It just means it is a relative improvement.

Another thing that can happen is that a transition to paleo may inadvertently remove an allergen or a food to which someone is particularly sensitive from the diet, producing improvements. For example, a person may have an undetected problem with wheat, and a paleo diet may produce relief since it necessarily eliminates wheat in most cases. But it could be that the very same improvements could have been experienced simply by eliminating wheat alone while continuing to include rice, beans, sugar, and dairy in the diet. But since the positive changes are attributed to paleo as a whole, the diet may become unnecessarily restrictive. And, unfortunately, as we'll see, since the trend in paleo seems to be for increasing restriction, eventually such a person may find that they reduce carbohydrates and other foods that really would be quite healthy for that particular person all because the person identifies with paleo.

Depending on the version of paleo that a person subscribes to, it *may* be sustainable. And, if it is and the person continues to enjoy their diet and lifestyle, that is great. There's no problem with that. However, many versions of paleo—particularly the ultra-restrictive versions that are becoming increasingly the norm—are *not* sustainable. They *may* confer short-term benefits, particularly if someone is transitioning from an unhealthy lifestyle and diet. However, the very qualities that make the restrictive diets beneficial in the short term are likely to produce problems in the long term.

One example of this is weight loss. Now, to be clear, as I've written about in other books, I do not perceive that weight loss is always or even often a good thing in and of itself. However, in some cases when people are extremely overweight, a person may feel much better after losing some weight. If subscribing to paleo seems to produce weight loss that is perceived as positive to an individual, that person may then strongly identify with paleo. And yet, continued adherence to a diet that produces weight loss may not be a great idea. Why? Because that weight loss *may* have come about as a result of calorie deficiency, and continued calorie deficiency, as I have detailed in other books, produces the symptoms of starvation, which are not desirable or pleasant. Unfortunately, these symptoms are rarely recognized for what they are these days, and so a lot of starving people keep searching for answers to their problems in the very thing that is producing the problems. In other words, they stick to paleo all the more rigidly, not recognizing that the rigidity of the particular interpretation of the diet they are adhering to is starving them.

The bottom line here is that *some* versions of the paleo diet are healthy and sustainable (though not necessarily more than a diet that also includes dairy, sugar, grain, and legumes), but many are not—at least not for everyone. And, just because someone experiences some perceived benefits from switching to a paleo diet initially does not mean that those benefits are all *because* of the diet. At the very least, even if the change in diet is responsible for some benefits, it may not be produced by the aspects of the diet that one imagines.

The Fallacy of the Paleo Foods Myth

The core of the paleo diet is the inclusion of "good" foods and the exclusion of "bad" foods. The criteria for inclusion or exclusion is the deceptively simple guide that good foods are those that mimic what our Paleolithic ancestors would have eaten while the bad foods are Neolithic inventions. In other words, good Paleolithic analogs include things like grass-fed beef, kale, and sweet potatoes while bad Neolithic inventions include grains, beans, sugar, and dairy.

The problem with this is just that it is arbitrary, unnecessarily restrictive, and naive. Here's why. The simple rules that guide paleo have allowed paleo to take on religious overtones. I'm not the only one who thinks so. In fact, this criticism has been leveled frequently enough that many of the paleo gurus, Sisson and Wolf included, have publicly defended the lifestyle/movement by declaring that it is *not* a religion. While there may not be a church of paleo, the zeal with which many adherents and gurus alike approach the subject—and the *disdain* with which they often speak of any *other* diet—stinks a lot like religious wars.

When a movement takes on religious overtones, it seems likely that the adherents have subscribed to a myth or two. In the case of paleo, one of the key myths is that paleo food is good while non-paleo food is bad.

But one of the problems with this myth is that the distinctions are, as I have written, arbitrary. Paleo analogs like grass-fed beef and kale are held to be perfect foods while dairy and grain are Neolithic evils. But the truth is that beef and kale are just as Neolithic as dairy and grain. Truly. Look it up.

I'm not the first one to level this criticism, of course. And so paleo enthusiasts are quick to counter that the paleo analogs are, well, *analogs* to paleo foods whereas dairy, grain, sugar, legumes, and the like have no counterpart in true Paleolithic diets. But, there are a few errors with this logic.

Short of a working time flux capacitor and a DeLorean or successfully thawing Caveman Lawyer, we can't know for certain what our Paleolithic ancestors actually ate. But we do have some clues. Depending on climate and season, our ancestors probably ate a wide variety of foods, including fish, small game like squirrels and rabbits, large game like elk or bear, berries, tubers, nuts, and seeds. In addition, there is mounting evidence that they also ate some wild grains and legumes as evidenced by fossil records and tools. In fact, there is good reason to believe that our Paleolithic ancestors regularly ate the stomach contents of their prey, which would have included grains and legumes as well as dairy in the case of nursing mammals. I can attest to the fact that at least some contemporary "wilderness enthusiasts" eat the "cheese" found in the stomachs of young mammals. So while grain, legumes, and dairy probably didn't make up the main part of our Paleolithic ancestors' diets, neither were they strictly avoided.

Along with stomach contents, there is good reason to believe that our Paleolithic ancestors also ate the actual stomachs, lungs, kidneys, eyeballs (which are actually delicious), brains, paws and hooves, and most of the rest of the animals that they consumed. The wilderness school where I stayed subjected its long-term students to periods of hunger so that they would try to fend for themselves. I was witness to people eating all kinds of things, including live frogs. And you can bet that when they were hungry, our Paleolithic ancestors did the same.

When it comes to plant foods, true Paleolithic fare was likely quite a bit different than the kale and sweet potatoes of modern paleo diets. In northern Wisconsin, we ate wild harvested nettle, tamarack leaves, and wild leeks. The tubers and roots that our Paleolithic ancestors ate were small and relatively bitter compared to modern, cultivated tubers and roots. And for the most part, the nuts and seeds that they ate were hard to come by—a lot harder than picking up a two pound bag of shelled and roasted nuts from Trader Joe's, at least—and they were generally smaller and more toxic than modern nuts. There are exceptions, of course, but most modern nuts have been bred to be larger and less toxic. So Grok probably wasn't shoving fistfuls of almonds in his mouth—he was eating a few wild apricot kernels at a time, more like.

In general, wild Paleolithic foods, like most wild foods today, were leaner, tougher, more bitter, more fibrous, and less palatable than cultivated foods today. And unless a person is eating a couple of frogs, an eyeball, a bit of stomach contents, a hoof, a wild carrot, a tiger nut, a crab apple, and some wild grape leaves for their sustenance, I doubt that person is *really* eating a diet that mimics a true Paleolithic diet.

Does that mean that the so-called paleo diet as practiced by many people today is inherently bad or unhealthy? Not necessarily. But the idea that the modern paleo diet has anything to do with real Paleolithic diets is absurd.

Some sophisticated paleo enthusiasts will counter that the purpose of the modern paleo diet is to avoid toxins in food. They claim that grains, legumes, dairy, sugar, and potatoes all contain harmful toxins that are best to be avoided. And that is true...sort of. But it's misleading.

The reality is that *all* foods contain toxins. Generally speaking, meats contain the fewest toxins, presumably because most animals are able to move as a defense system whereas plants use toxins to defend themselves—making themselves unpalatable. But the notion that grains, legumes, dairy, sugar, and potatoes contain toxins *more than* most other foods is simply not true.

Paleo staples like cabbage, kale, sweet potatoes, and carrots all contain cyanide compounds that are potentially toxic to humans. When the body detoxifies them, they convert into substances that block iodine uptake in the thyroid, which can produce endocrine disorders.

And, in fact, many of the substances found in fruits and vegetables that are touted as being health-promoting only provide the health benefits in *small* amounts. When eaten in large amounts, their toxic effects can begin to manifest. So chowing down on six pounds of kale a day (like you would need to do to meet Loren Cordain's advice) isn't such a great idea. In other words, more isn't always better.

Interestingly, however, most wild plant foods are tougher, more bitter, more sour, and more pungent exactly because they are more concentrated sources of these substances that are healthful in small amounts and possibly toxic in large amounts. Cultivated plant foods have been bred to have fewer of these toxins. In part, that is what makes them more palatable.

As we'll explore together throughout the book, many of the foods excluded by most paleo enthusiasts do, in fact, have some toxic substances. But as we'll also see, the actual dangers have been overstated, and it is not clear that the dangers of those substances are any worse than those of the paleo-approved foods. In fact, many refined grains, sugar, and dairy actually contain *fewer* known toxins than broccoli and sweet potatoes.

Hopefully you can see that the actual story of the true Paleolithic diet is a bit more complex than we've been led to believe. How many of the bitter, sour, fibrous, and pungent plant foods were our ancestors actually eating? What are the effects of eating stomach contents and brains as well as, one would assume, a fair amount of dirt on health? And does the modern paleo diet actually mimic the real Paleolithic diet?

Of course, I am not suggesting that one *should* strive to mimic the true Paleolithic diet. However, if the premise of the paleo diet is that our ancestors were healthier because of what they ate (or didn't eat), it seems worthwhile to investigate whether the proposed paleo diet actually lives up to the hype. And after a little bit of investigation, I'd say that it doesn't seem to.

The Paleolithic Perfection Myth

Next, let's consider whether the notion that our Paleolithic ancestors really were so perfectly healthy is actually true. After all, this assumption is at the heart of the paleo diet argument. If our Paleolithic ancestors weren't truly as pristinely healthy as we have been led to believe, then it certainly undermines the argument that their diet was the reason for that supposedly perfect health.

The assertion is that Paleolithic humans never suffered from diabetes, cardiovascular disease, cancer, Alzheimer's, Parkinson's, or any other ill health is, in truth, a giant load of horse shit. Or mammoth shit, if you prefer. While it is certainly possible that Grok and company were tall, strong, virile, and always healthy, the truth is: *we don't know*. We don't know because we're talking about a *very* long time ago. There are no written records from the time, and the archeological evidence is thin. Why? Again, because we're talking about a very long time ago, and in general, under most conditions found on Earth, stuff decomposes within 10,000 years.

What all of that means is that, like I stated earlier, short of a time machine or some other extraordinary means, much of what we think we know about that time and human behavior at the time is guesswork.

With that said, some of the best guesswork at present suggests that the transition between Paleolithic and Neolithic eras was marked by tradeoffs when it comes to human health. For example, according to John Lawrence Angel, who was a biological anthropologist and the father of modern paleopathology, humans living in the late Paleolithic (between 30,000 and 9,000 B.C.E.) had median lifespans of 35 (male) and 30 (female). But in the late Neolithic (between 5,000 and 3,000 B.C.E.), the median lifespans were 33 and 29, suggesting that something during that time led to decreased lifespan. Some claim that median lifespan is not a useful value because it factors in infant mortality. However, it seems to me that it *is* a useful metric precisely because it includes infant mortality. If we want to know the overall health of a group of people, knowing how successful they are in reproducing and having their children live into adulthood is a useful bit of information.

As you can see, the best guesses suggest that the transition to agriculture saw a small but significant drop in median lifespan. However, a thousand years after the late Neolithic, median lifespans *exceeded* those of the Paleolithic, and they have continued to rise until present. So overall, median lifespan doesn't make a strong argument for or against agriculture.

What is, perhaps, more significant is that we are told that remains from the Paleolithic period show that the bones were strong and healthy, the teeth were free of cavities, and the pelvic inlet depth was large. Some argue that a large pelvic inlet depth makes birth easier, and it is argued that some very few modern women still exhibit large pelvic inlet depths when eating traditional diets free of large amounts of grains and legumes. Whether or not this claim is true, I cannot validate. But what I can report is that Angel published a report in which he stated that the pelvic inlet depth index percent in the late Paleolithic was 97.7 and that it decreased in the Neolithic to 76.6, increasing only slightly over time to an average of 82 today among white North Americans and Europeans.

We are also told that in the Neolithic, bones began to exhibit weakness and deformity and that teeth first began to exhibit cavities. The claim is that grains and legumes created this change. And *this* is why paleo diet enthusiasts (whether they know it or not) argue in favor of excluding grains and legumes from the diet.

So far, it would seem that perhaps the paleo advocates are correct. Maybe we really should exclude legumes and grains because clearly they caused poor health in Neolithic people.

But hold on just a second because that's quite a leap. All we know is that *possibly* at least *some* Paleolithic people had better bones, teeth, and pelvic inlet depths than Neolithic people. But even if that is the case, we simply don't know *why* that might be. Could it be due to grain and legume consumption in the Neolithic? It *could* be. But could it be due to very different reasons? Yup. It sure could be.

What could some of those other reasons be? Well, it could have been due to increasing population density or diseases increased by the practice of animal husbandry (things like chicken pox and smallpox or tetanus, for example). Also, although nomadism in the Paleolithic is associated with increased death, the tendency toward sedentarism in the Neolithic may have had a tendency to subtly reduce the quality of the food, or it may have exposed people to toxins found in a particular area for longer periods of time. These are merely guesses. But then again, so is the guess that the changes in health were brought about simply because of the introduction of grain and legumes (and dairy and sugar, apparently).

For another thing, it *does* seem true that there are health consequences of relying heavily upon improperly prepared whole grains and legumes as a major source of food. And yes, it is reasonable to believe that the Neolithic saw a major increase in these foods in the human diet. And that *may* have had a negative impact on health in some respects. However, that isn't enough to indict grains and legumes. After all, some of the people who are considered to be the healthiest and longest-lived today, the Okinawans, have a traditional diet that, on average, consists of 150 grams of rice and 70 grams of beans daily. Do the Okinawans have reduced pelvic inlet depths as a result? Maybe. But then again, maybe not. We just don't know, and the evidence against grains and beans with sweeping generalizations is naive and immature.

One of the other things that I find fascinating when claims are made about the pristine health of the

Paleolithic people is that no mention is made of the dramatic increase in median lifespan since then and the implications of that when it comes to disease. Furthermore, infant mortality is generally not discussed in terms of the implications of how that might skew the development of diseases and sickness within a population.

In the late Paleolithic, the median lifespan for men was 35. There were, most likely, plenty of people who lived into their 60s. However, not *nearly* as many as do today. In fact, the percentage of the population that is older than 60 is presently growing, meaning that not only are people living longer, but the entire population is now older than ever before. When we talk about the diseases of civilization that are pinned on agriculture, we're mostly talking about things like diabetes, cardiovascular disease, cancer, Alzheimer's, etc. Guess what the number one risk factor for all of these diseases is. It's advanced age. In other words, when the world population gets older, as it is presently, it is expected that there will be greater rates of these diseases. Meanwhile, a younger population such as might have been found during the Paleolithic would be expected to have far fewer incidences.

Infant mortality may also play a role in the rates of disease as well. It is expected that not only were natural infant death rates considerably higher in the Paleolithic, rates of infanticide were also higher. Of course, we cannot know why babies died or why they were killed, but we can speculate that the most susceptible may have died and those who were deemed sickly or undesirable may have been killed. And, it is reasonable to expect that under such circumstances, the rates of disease in adults might be lower as a result. Meanwhile, present day infant mortality rates are relatively extremely low. But it *could* be that reduced infant mortality rates may contribute to greater rates of disease in adults.

As I mentioned earlier, the transition from Paleolithic to Neolithic lifestyles seems to have been a tradeoff. On the one hand, for reasons that are unknown (that *could* have had to do with dietary changes, but just as well could have been due to other factors), Neolithic people *seem* to have exhibited worsening bone and tooth health compared to the remains of Paleolithic people that have been studied. But on the other hand, there is pretty good evidence that humans have done quite well since the transition. After all, the population has ballooned from just a handful of people scattered around the globe to over 7 *billion* people. Median lifespans have increased. And, truth be told, it would seem that the claim that rates of disease have actually increased is unproven. As I have pointed out, it could be simply that more people survive into adulthood and more people live to be older than during Paleolithic times, creating the *illusion* of greater rates of disease.

All in all, I have yet to come across a truly convincing argument that Paleolithic people were the specimens of health and vitality that we are led to believe by paleo diet enthusiasts. They may have been, but we just don't know that to be the case. And the claim that foods introduced in larger quantities in the Neolithic period are the cause of the supposed decline in health is speculative at best.

Phytic Acid

Phytic acid is one of those things that the paleo advocates like to harp on about. In case you're not familiar, phytic acid is a substance found in some of the foods that are generally strictly forbidden in paleo diets such as grains and legumes. One of the things that phytic acid does is bind together with minerals such as calcium, magnesium, and zinc, keeping them in storage in the seed (grains and legumes are seeds) until the seed germinates. Viable seeds (meaning they haven't been subjected to heat or age or other factors that would prevent them from germinating) will contain enough of an enzyme called phytase in order to deactivate phytic acid, liberating the minerals that the seed will then use to begin growing into a new plant.

The primary objection to phytic acid in foods is that since it binds to minerals, it makes those minerals unavailable to humans. And, to be sure, that can cause some problems. For example, the minerals zinc and copper need to be kept in a favorable ratio in the human body since each is important and they compete within the body. So if one is too high or too low, that will cause problems. Normally these minerals are found in the right ratio in foods. And, in fact, they are usually found in the right ratio in many legumes. However, since legumes contain phytic acid and phytic acid selectively binds to zinc but not copper, eating these foods can produce a mineral imbalance. But, frankly, it's only likely to happen if one relies heavily upon improperly prepared grains and legumes in the diet. In moderation, it's probably not a problem.

The paleo argument against phytic acid makes it sound like a big deal. I've actually seen headlines claiming, "Phytic acid in grains is killing you." But these claims are unfounded. In fact, all evidence is that phytic acid binds to minerals, but that is probably the worst of it. Claims that it can cross into the blood are unsubstantiated since I do not know of a single study that demonstrates that happening.

Eating large amounts of phytic acid is linked to tooth demineralization and may be connected with bone problems, but only because it prevents absorption of the minerals in the foods containing phytic acid. There is no evidence that phytic acid foods can actually pull minerals from the body. Rather, it's just that if one eats large amounts of phytic acid foods, the bioavailable mineral content of the foods eaten is relatively low. This can be easily corrected by simply eating fewer foods containing phytic acid and more foods containing bioavailable minerals. That's really not that big of a deal.

One of the reasons that beans are traditionally soaked and sprouted before cooking is that the process reduces the phytic acid content. The longer the sprouting process, the greater the reduction in phytic acid. So for those who really want to eat *lots* of beans, proper preparation can make a big difference.

One of the possible reasons (among others) that some grains have been refined to have their bran removed is that the phytic acid content is in the bran. So removing the bran removes the phytic acid content. Granted, that also removes most of the minerals. However, it is possible that phytic acid in a food may bind with the minerals of the other foods eaten with the phytic acid. For example, brown rice eaten with beef *may* bind to the zinc in the beef, making it unavailable. So eating white rice or other refined grains may be yet another traditional way in which people have made use of the energy in grains while avoiding some of the possible negatives when eaten in large amounts.

Fermentation also reduces phytic acid. Weston A. Price, the famous dentist who studied the dental health of traditional cultures around the globe, found that sourdough bread made from freshly ground whole wheat was an excellent food for restoring dental health. Remember that phytic acid is associated with dental decay. However, Price found that a long fermentation process makes whole wheat an excellent source of nutrition, including minerals needed for healthy teeth and jaw development.

Ironically, although many paleo advocates demonize phytic acid, foods like nuts, seeds, chocolate (dark or raw, of course!), and coffee are often staples among paleo enthusiasts. I say this is ironic because these paleo-approved foods contain some of the *highest* levels of phytic acid of all foods—much higher than grains or legumes in most cases. Of course, few people eat cashews as a staple as they might brown rice and beans, but then again, Brazil nuts or raw chocolate (cacao) have nearly twice the phytic acid of brown rice by weight. And, considering the amount of coffee, chocolate, and nuts some paleo enthusiasts consume, it turns out to be a lot. But, amazingly, they often claim that they are benefiting from their pure, ancestral diet. Which just might mean that maybe phytic acid isn't ast big of a deal as it's been made out to be.

The truth seems to be that large amounts of phytic acid eaten regularly may produce undesirable effects for some people. And reducing the amount of phytic acid that one eats is probably a sensible thing to do. I don't recommend eating brown rice and unsprouted beans along with handfuls of sesame seeds and gallons of coffee and hot chocolate as your staples. That's probably a bad idea.

But on the other hand, many non-paleo diets that include grains and maybe even some legumes probably have lower phytic acid levels than many popular paleo diets. Remember, white rice has negligible amounts of phytic acid. So the phytic acid argument is really a fail when it comes to paleo.

Lectins

Next, let's look at lectins, which are another one of those substances that are demonized by many paleo proponents. It turns out that *most* lectins, which are a certain type of protein found in plants and animals, are actually either neutral or even healthy when it comes to the food that humans eat. The lectins that are of most concern are called agglutinins, and, not surprisingly, agglutinins are found primarily in grains and legumes, which further supports the paleo distaste for them. But these villainous lectins are also found in nightshades such as potatoes, tomatoes, pepper, and eggplant, which is why many paleo enthusiasts shun nightshade foods. And they may also be found in dairy and in eggs, though it is not clear if they are only found when the dairy animals or poultry are fed grain and legumes. Neither is it clear why paleo enthusiasts give dairy the cold shoulder but eggs get a free pass when it comes to the lectin issue.

Some are absolutely fanatical in their zeal to prevent us from ingesting these toxic substances. And, to be clear, they *are* toxic. But it's not *that* big of a deal for *most* people. Sure, some people are highly sensitive and should avoid them. But for most, it's not like these agglutinins are going to kill, *despite* the fact that Dave Asprey, the Bulletproof Executive guy who is, arguably, a paleo guru, wrote an entire article about the dangers of agglutinins. He actually made the claim that, and I quote, "[o]nly a few raw kidney beans can kill you because [of] the naturally occurring lectins." Well, sorry to burst his bubble (okay, not really sorry at all), but back in my raw vegan days, I actually ate more than a few raw kidney beans. I must have eaten a cup of them all at once. (And yes, they do taste rather horrid, in case you were wondering. And no, I really cannot explain what possessed me to eat them.) I *did* end up with some mild nausea for an hour. I did *not* die. Not even close. I didn't even vomit.

Is it true that raw kidney beans contain a toxic lectin? Yes. Is it fatally toxic in moderate amounts? Not generally. There is a report of an ill-fated "healthy eating day" at a U.S. hospital that occurred in 1988. The staff cafeteria served up some (apparently undercooked) kidney beans and an hour later, while the staff was participating in a lecture, several women began to vomit. But no one died. Why? Because for most people in moderate amounts, they aren't *fatally* toxic. They'll just make a person feel unwell and maybe vomit. So some people in the paleo crowd are spreading misinformation.

The other thing about these supposedly fatally toxic (but not really) lectins is that most of them are deactivated by sufficient heat. In other words, cooking deactivates them. That is why *thoroughly* cooked kidney beans, despite their ridiculously high toxic lectin content, don't make people sick.

According to Mat Lalonde, a Harvard University lecturer with a keen interest in nutrition and paleo, there are only a few lectins that are actually of concern, and the only one people are likely to eat is found in peanuts. The peanut lectin survives some cooking and can actually get into the bloodstream where it may cause immune reactions. So for those who are sensitive to peanuts, it might be best to avoid them. But then again, plenty of people seem to have no problem. So there you go. Consider lectins a major fail for paleo.

Insulin

Another one of the things that many paleo advocates run on about is insulin, which is an important anabolic (meaning tissue building) hormone that occurs naturally in the body. Insulin does *many* things, but one of the things it is most famous for is moving energy and protein from the bloodstream into cells. That is a very important function without which we'd probably all drop dead pretty quickly since cells need energy all the time.

Paleo gurus like Mark Sisson have all but declared war on insulin. Sisson advises in his *Primal Blueprint* that we should strive to eat between 50 and 100 grams of carbohydrates per day (or maybe less) so that we can "minimize insulin production" because in his view, insulin is bad.

Sisson describes insulin merely as a means for storing "excess nutrients." In his view, almost everyone is eating too much, and insulin only exists to keep us from dying from our gluttony by storing all that excess sugar as fat in the body. His description misled me and has misled many people into starving themselves of carbohydrates and possibly calories as well. He also indicts dairy almost exclusively because of its insulinogenic properties, causing people to fear dairy.

But he's wrong. Insulin doesn't exist merely to keep "toxic" (his word) glucose (blood sugar) out of the blood, moving it into adipose tissue instead. That is not true. As I have already written, insulin helps to get nutrients into the cells where they are needed. *That* is what it does. And if everything is going well at the cellular level, insulin production is absolutely wonderful because that insulin keeps feeding the cells to keep them (and you) alive.

The problem isn't with insulin. The problem is when cellular respiration is impaired, and the cells *block* insulin as a way of preventing excess input from harming the cell. There are plenty of things that might harm cellular respiration, but insulin response to eating carbohydrates (or protein) isn't likely to be one of them. And if a person is experiencing insulin resistance, that most likely signifies a problem with cellular respiration, so reducing carbohydrates and insulin production may work as a stopgap measure in the short run, but it doesn't necessarily address the underlying problem, which is poorly functioning cellular respiration.

Many paleo gurus (Sisson may be the worst of them) have used distorted information and strangely contorted logic to persuade people that cells should be fueled exclusively by ketones, which are derived from fat. Using this logic, Sisson and others suggest that dramatically reducing carbohydrate intake and insulin secretion is the ideal state. But they are overlooking the fact that, despite their claims, the body will go to great lengths to fuel cells using glucose. In fact, no matter what, the brain *always* requires glucose. Except for the most extreme circumstances (which we'll address shortly), the body will continue to produce glucose to fuel *all* cells, even if it has to convert protein to glucose—even if it has to break down muscle to convert muscle protein to glucose. We're talking about terrifically inefficient processes that the body will go through just to produce glucose to fuel cells. Why? Because it would seem that the body actually prefers glucose—a.k.a. sugar.

Leptin

Next on the list of paleo enemy hormones is leptin. Paleo advocates are often quick to admit that leptin is a relatively new discovery about which very little is actually known. But, unfortunately, that doesn't stop most paleo proponents from 'splainin' leptin to us as the hormone that fat people make more of because they eat too many freaking carbohydrates. They explain that leptin resistance occurs because of overeating those devilish (but delicious) carbohydrates that are found in things like potatoes, legumes, grains, fruits, and sugar, and that fat people are always leptin resistant. We are led to believe that fat people are fat just because of them darn carbs.

The paleo leptin story dovetails nicely with the paleo insulin story. (Incidentally, as I write this, I am now remembering the other low-carb paleo zealot who has convinced millions of people that carbohydrates and insulin are the devil—Gary Taubes.) Unfortunately, like the insulin story, the leptin story defies reality.

It is *really* easy to disprove the simplified paleo leptin story. All I have to do is point out that there are billions of skinny people all over the world who eat *mostly* carbohydrates, including *all* of the stuff the paleo crowd have written off as the handiwork of Satan himself. I mean, really, call to mind for a moment the image of a die-hard fruitarian who gorges on sugar-laden fruit and fruit juices all day long. Or what about a Chinese person eating a traditional diet with tons of white rice? What about that guy you know who is always going on about how he lost 100 pounds eating a vegan diet (you know, the sort that is *all* carbohydrates)? Heck, there are lots of people in the Ray Peat crowd who guzzle white sugar syrup, orange juice, and milk all day. And what all these stereotypes have in common is that *they are not fat*. If anything, they are often *too* thin.

Sorry, but the leptin story is another paleo fail.

Even the guy who co-discovered leptin can't agree. That guy, Rudolph Leibel, a medical doctor who is presently working at Columbia University, has done some elaborate tests that demonstrate that by and large people don't get fat because of what they eat or how much they eat. He showed that the more people eat, the faster they burn calories, and the less people eat, the slower they burn calories. And it doesn't particularly matter whether those calories are from grass-fed, wild, local, hand-killed venison or Krispy Kreme. *There are different mechanisms at work in getting fat.* Leptin may play a role, but it ain't the one the paleo crowd is telling us.

Low Carb

While we're on a roll with these hormones that supposedly make people fat and sick solely because people are eating too many carbohydrates, let's look at the advice that generally comes out of it, which is: eat a low-carbohydrate diet to be trim, athletic, healthy, sexy, and wealthy. Okay, I made up the bit about becoming wealthy from eating low carb since, let's face it, them carbs is cheap compared to all that grass-fed meat and kale you've got to eat instead.

It's ironic that low carb has become conflated with paleo. I say it's ironic for two reasons. For one thing, Loren Cordain, the guy who turned paleo into a celebrity with the publication of *The Paleo Diet,*™ actually advises people to eat between 35 and 45 percent of their calories from carbohydrates. (Granted, he does suggest that those calories come mostly from low-starch and low-sugar foods, so I'm not sure how on earth anyone could actually accomplish that goal since that would require eating about 6 *pounds* of kale a day.) For a person who needs 3000 calories per day, that means eating between 1050 and 1350 calories from carbohydrates, which is a *far cry* from Sisson's claim that eating more than 150 grams of carbohydrates in a day will lead to "insidious weight gain."

The second reason I say it's ironic is that there are *very few* known examples of traditional diets that are actually low in carbohydrates where we define "low in carbohydrates" by the conventional standards used in most paleo crowds these days, which means *less than 200 grams of carbohydrates per day*. And, in fact, there are examples of modern hunter-gatherer diets in which the people obtain as much as *85 percent* of their calories from carbohydrates—and not just non-starchy, non-sugary carbohydrates. For the record, those people have traditionally had low incidences of disease and haven't been notably fat.

Does low-carbohydrate eating suit some people some of the time? Sure. Of course it does. But just because some people feel good eating low carb for a while doesn't mean that *everyone* should or that *most* will necessarily thrive on such a diet *long term*. Again, there are *very few* known traditional diets in which people have eaten so few carbohydrates. Low-carb paleo enthusiasts may dismiss that evidence, suggesting that all that means is that the majority of humans are and have been addicted to carbohydrates and suffer as a result. But that's insane since there are innumerable examples of individuals and entire cultures that are and have been quite healthy *and happy* eating carbohydrates.

Are some people better suited to eating carbohydrates than others? Probably. It turns out that some people secrete more starch-digesting enzymes than others. But it turns out that *all* humans secrete starch-digesting enzymes. So while your neighbor may be more inclined to eat only 35 percent of his calories from carbohydrates, your other neighbor may be predisposed to functioning better with 85 percent of calories coming from carbohydrates. There's some room for variation, but by and large, *most* humans seem to have evolved in the context of eating a significant portion of calories from carbohydrates.

Low-carbohydrate diets have been associated with euthyroid sick syndrome (low thyroid hormone levels), disturbed cortisol patterns, and...low leptin and insulin. What are the effects? Fatigue, mood disturbance, insomnia, hair loss, brain fog, and more. For some people, it takes longer to reach this state on a low-carbohydrate diet than others, which is why some people become low-carb zealots for a few weeks or months or years while other people crash and burn right away. But in the long run, there are not a lot of reports of people who thrive on low-carbohydrate diets in the long term. Most have to at least cycle in some high-carbohydrate days. And, really, there's a lot that we don't know about why some people are able to do low-carb eating for a longer term. It could be that there is a genetic component that allows some people to do it while most cannot.

To reiterate, I am fully aware that not *all* paleo advocates promote low-carb diets. However, this criticism is valid and necessary because in *many* popular paleo crowds, paleo very definitely *is* synonymous with low-carbohydrate eating.

Keto

Since we've covered low-carbohydrate diets, let's also look at the variant, which are ketogenic diets. Although keto is a minor subset of paleo, it's significant enough to warrant some attention. Sisson, Moore, Phinney, Volek, and other low-carb gurus who are at least strongly associated with paleo advocate for ketogenic diets to greater or lesser extents. They promote the idea that ketones are the natural and preferred fuel for human cells, and that glucose is inferior and harmful. As a result, a lot of people seem to have gotten the idea that ketosis is the ideal.

Ketosis is the state in which the body burns fat for fuel, producing ketone bodies. Ketones can be used by most cells in place of glucose. The exception are brain cells which still require at least half glucose in order to survive. Nutritional ketosis—a ketogenic state induced intentionally through diet—does have some limited therapeutic applications. Notably, ketosis has been shown to help in *some* cases of epilepsy. However, just because ketosis is *sometimes* useful in the short term for very specific conditions does not mean that it is always preferable.

In my view, the simplest way to refute the ketosis-is-best-for-everyone-all-the-time argument is to investigate whether a) the body seems to actually prefer ketosis and b) whether inducing ketosis within the food context in which our ancestors evolved is reasonably easy.

In order to produce nutritional ketosis, carbohydrate *and* protein intake has to be *very low*. That is because the body will convert all carbohydrates *and* any excess protein to glucose if given a chance. In fact, it will even convert *fat* to glucose if necessary. (Remember, the brain requires at least half glucose all the time. So if dietary carbohydrates and protein are inadequate, the body will be forced to make an inefficient conversion of fat to glucose to keep the brain alive.) There are some modern tricks that can be used to allow for a *slightly* elevated carbohydrate and protein intake by including medium-chain triglyceride oil (derived from coconut or palm oil, usually), which increases ketone production. Different ketosis gurus have different recommendations, but generally for a 3000-calorie diet, protein intake will be around 100 grams and carbohydrate intake will be less than 50, meaning that 2400 calories have to be gotten from fat. For *most* people, that is not appetizing. That amounts to eating a third of a pound of lean beef, a carrot, and a *full stick* of butter for a meal. So based on the amount of effort involved and the lack of appetite that most will have for such a diet, I don't think that ketosis seems to be the preferred state for the body.

Next, let's consider that in *most* environments, there is no natural source of food that would facilitate a ketogenic diet. True, in *some* tropical environments there exists a relative abundance of foods like coconuts, which could allow for a person who is dedicated to ketosis to achieve and maintain the state. But by and large, most foods just don't provide anything approaching the ratios of fat to everything else necessary. I cannot think of a single animal whose composition would allow one to enter ketosis by eating the whole animal. Even seals, which are relatively fat, are only about 14 percent fat. So I think it is darn near impossible to make an argument that the natural environment implies that ketosis is the preferred state.

The Good, The Bad, The Ugly

Generally, there is much that is good about paleo as long as we view it in the least restrictive sense. A non-restrictive approach to paleo includes adequate (but not excessive) quality protein, good fats, and quality carbohydrates. And all of that food is nutritionally dense in that it contains lots of nutrients. And, furthermore, paleo excludes stuff like hydrogenated vegetable oil, artificial sweeteners, high-fructose corn syrup, artificial colors, seitan, and soy protein isolate—things that really don't make for good food and are probably best left out of *most* diets *most* of the time. It is certainly possible to eat a healthy and sustainable diet that fits within this definition of paleo.

But are the benefits that can be had by switching to the paleo diet *only* available with a diet that also eliminates milk, cheese, maple syrup, cane sugar, white rice, potatoes, pasta, and other foods that, for many people, are actually *perfectly healthy and nutritious*? By eliminating these foods rather arbitrarily, many people will experience unnecessary stress and potentially some nutritional deficiencies.

The idea that it is possible to experience nutritional deficiencies on a diet as supposedly perfect as the paleo diet is generally offensive to the adherents in the same way that most vegans are in denial about the nutritional deficiencies that can happen on the supposedly perfect plant-based diet. But despite the belief and denial, the reality is that food restrictions that eliminate entire categories of *real* food do come with an increased risk of creating nutritional deficiencies. Admittedly, nutritional deficiencies on an *inclusive* paleo diet will probably be few, but it's still worth considering why one should eliminate real foods that are abundant sources of nutrition if there is no *actual* negative reaction to those foods.

For example, the reality is that dairy is *the best* source of calcium in most people's diets. True, if one eats a can or two of sardines each day it is possible to obtain enough, but really, are you doing that? Bone broth turns out *not* to be a great source of calcium, and even if it were, are you *really* going to prepare and consume *that much* bone broth? This then leaves you with the same calcium sources as the vegans who are *notoriously* deficient in calcium. Those leafy greens that are touted as good sources of calcium have a bioavailability of about 35 percent (give or take, depending on the vegetable), which means you'd have to eat *way more kale* than you're actually going to eat in order to eat enough calcium.

Perhaps the most common nutritional deficiency with many paleo diets is a *calorie* deficiency. Most people these days cannot fathom that such a thing even exists, but, in fact, it does. It's called starvation—or semi-starvation if the S-word is too blunt. I'm pretty sure that our Paleolithic ancestors knew the tremendous importance of eating enough just the same as those of us huddled around a campfire in the middle of a northern Wisconsin winter knew that without enough food, we were going to feel a whole lot worse. In fact, I'm willing to bet that the same ancestral knowledge about the importance of eating enough was passed down from generation to generation all the way up until a few generations ago. That's why many of us had parents or grandparents who knew that the solution to *any* problem was food— because a lot of the time that's true!

But lately we've lost that wisdom. We've been told time and time again that when it comes to calories, less is more. So any dietary change that allows us to eat fewer calories while feeling full comes as a godsend. In fact, that is precisely one of the qualities of the paleo diet that is so appealing to many people; it serves as a short-term weight loss diet because due to its (generally) moderate protein, moderate (to high) fat, and high-fiber whole foods nature, people transitioning from eating more processed foods will almost always end up eating fewer calories. If one has a lot of stored energy (typically in adipose tissue), then it is *possible* that the transition will be a smooth one and that it will be perceived entirely as positive.

However, sooner or later, for most people who are eating a calorie-deficient diet, the effects will be felt. And those effects aren't pleasant because chronic calorie deficiency is actually the ultimate nutritional deficiency.

It leads to anxiety, insomnia, fatigue, irritability, digestive problems, arthritis, and symptoms too numerous to list.

Of course, calorie deficiency isn't going to happen in every case, but any dietary restriction increases the likelihood of calorie deficiency, and I'd wager that it happens more often on a paleo diet than most people are aware. Combine paleo with low carb, which is common, and you've got an even more restrictive diet that increases the likelihood of deficiency even more.

But you've got to ask yourself, "What's the point?" Sure, anyone who genuinely has a problem with a particular food should probably avoid that food for as long as they have a problem with it. For example, one of my best friends from high school had (and likely still has) a severe allergy to legumes. In fact, eating peanuts or lentils put him at risk of going into anaphylactic shock. So I wouldn't ever recommend that such a person should go feast on hummus and refried beans. Neither would I suggest that someone with Celiac disease should eat seitan.

But the thing is, *most* people don't have these problems. Sure, it does seem to be true that gliadin (the problematic protein in gluten) is relatively hard to digest because of its complexity. But does that mean that it is harmful to most people? Not really. If someone has blood sugar control problems, it is sensible for that person to be careful (at least temporarily) with sugar consumption. But does that mean that sugar is harmful for *everyone*? Nope. And just because some people are lactose intolerant doesn't mean that everyone should avoid it.

The truth is that *all* food is toxic in some fashion. But ultimately, I suspect that fear of food and rigid mindsets are probably far more toxic.

In the end, as in the beginning, I don't care what you eat. And I respect that only you can find out what is right for you. But I do invite you to question any belief that says that it is best to avoid entire categories of food just because Mark Sisson or Rob Wolf or Art De Vany or your zealot friend says they are bad. Check it out for yourself. Use some good logic. Notice that the high rates of diseases pinned on dairy, potatoes, grains, and beans have all escalated in the past hundred years while those foods have been staples for people worldwide for *thousands* of years. The paleo story just doesn't *quite* add up.

Yes, some people will do best to avoid certain foods. And yes, some "foods" such as partially hydrogenated soybean oil are probably not good for most people. And, sure, eating *mostly* real, lightly processed foods, including meats, vegetables, fruits, and so forth is probably good advice *in general* most of the time—though not all of the time since sometimes people who are calorie deficient just need to eat a lot of food, and processed food affords that possibility. But none of that means that paleo is the right diet for everyone.

Don't be afraid of food. Especially don't be afraid of food that helps you to feel good. If eating "forbidden" foods helps you to sleep better, have more energy, and have a more stable mood and optimistic outlook, maybe that's a good thing. Remember, no matter what diet you want to champion, it is possible to find evidence to support the claims. You can find long-lived, healthy, happy people eating a wide variety of diets ranging from mostly meat to mostly fruit to mostly grain to mostly dairy and everything else.

Does diet matter? Probably. But the more I research, the more I suspect that it matters a lot less than most people think. It seems to me that if a particular food makes one sick it is best to avoid that food—at least for a while. And eating *mostly* real food that is lightly processed is probably *mostly* a good idea (though, as I wrote a moment ago, highly processed foods often have good therapeutic value). Eating *enough* is an oft-overlooked factor that plays an important role in health. But cutting out food groups because of ideology and because someone told you a story about how Grok was always healthy and strong turns out not to be the greatest idea.

Here's wishing you good eating, good health, and a good life—at least as best as it can be for you.

Get My Future Books FREE

If you enjoyed this book (Hey, if you made it this far it couldn't have been that bad), you'll probably enjoy many of my other books about health and wellness. And you can get all my new releases in health and wellness for free by signing up for my mailing list at www.joeylotthealth.com. It's simple, it's free, and it's totally honest and legitimate. Nothing scammy or spammy or anything else like that (i.e., I won't be trying to sell you The 7 Dirty Underground Top Secret Weird Tricks for Rock Hard Abs or Young Living Oils). It's just about free books for those who appreciate my work, because I appreciate YOU. Simple as that.

Connect With Me

I welcome your questions, comments, and feedback of any kind. Please feel free to email me at joeylott@gmail.com. I am now receiving so many emails that I cannot always reply to every one. I do read them all, and I do my best to reply to as many as possible. For the benefit of others, I may choose to publish my response to your email on my blog or in book format. I will maintain your privacy and anonymity if I choose to publish my response.

Connect With Me

My sincere goal in writing is to share something that may be of value to you. And I endeavor to do so while keeping the costs low for readers. The success of my books and my ability to reach other readers who may benefit from my books depends in large part on having lots of thoughtful, honest reviews written about my work. You would do me a great favor if you would please take a moment to generously write a review of this book at Amazon.com. This will only take a few minutes of your time, and you will be helping me a great deal. I sure would appreciate it.

About the Author

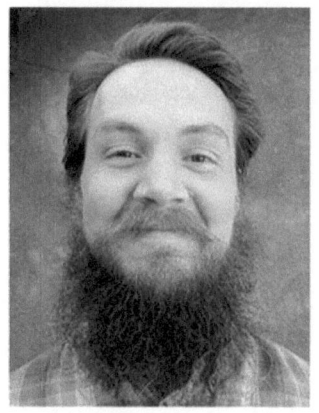

"The secret to happiness is to let go of everything - see through every assumption."

Beginning at a young age Joey Lott experienced intensifying anxiety. For several decades he lived with restrictive eating disorders, obsessions, compulsions, and an inescapable fear. By the time he was 30 years old he was physically sick, emotionally volatile, and mentally obsessed with keeping any and all unwanted thoughts and experiences at bay.

At this time Lott was living on a futon mattress in a tiny cabin in the woods. He was so sick that he could barely move. He was deeply depressed and hopeless. All this despite doing all the "right" things such as years of meditation, yoga, various "perfect" diets, clean air, and pure water.

Just when things were at their most dire, a crack appeared in the conceptual world that had formerly been mistaken for reality. By peering into this crack and underneath all the assumptions that had been unquestioned up to that moment, Lott began a great undoing. The revelation of this undoing is that reality is utterly simple, ever-present, seamless, and indivisible.

Lott's books provide a glimpse into the seamless, simple, and joyous nature of reality, offering a glimpse through the crack in conceptual worlds. Whether writing about the ultimate non-dual nature of reality, eating disorders, stress, disease, or any other subject, he offers the invitation to look at things differently, leaving behind the old, out-grown, painful limitations we have used to bind ourselves in suffering. And then, he welcomes you home to the effortless simplicity of yourself as you are.

Not sure where to begin? Pick up a copy of Lott's most popular book, *You're Trying Too Hard*, which strips away all the concepts that keep us searching for a greater, more spiritual, more peaceful life or self.

www.ingramcontent.com/pod-product-compliance
Lightning Source LLC
Chambersburg PA
CBHW050517290526
45786CB00007B/2600